Personal Information

Name:	Date of Birth:

Address:

Mobile Telephone:

Home Telephone:

Email:

Blood Group:

Weight:

Height:

Doctor's Information

Name:	Medications:

Address:

Email:

Mobile Telephone:

Emergency Contact

Name:	Relationship:

Address:

Email:

Mobile Telephone:

Understanding Blood Pressure Readings

What do your blood pressure numbers mean?

The only way to know if you have high blood pressure (HBP, or hypertension) is to have your blood pressure tested. Understanding your results is key to controlling high blood pressure.

Healthy and unhealthy blood pressure ranges
Learn what's considered normal,

as recommended by the American Heart Association.

Blood Pressure Category	Systolic mm Hg (upper number)		Diastolic mm Hg (lower number)
Normal	Less Than 120	&	Less Than 80
Elevated	120-129	&	Less Than 80
High Blood Pressure (hypertension) Stage 1	130-139	Or	80-89
High Blood Pressure (hypertension) Stage 2	140 Or Higher	Or	90 Or Higher
Hypertensive Crisis (Consult your doctor Immediately)	Higher Than 180	&/Or	Higher Than 120

Blood pressure categories

The five blood pressure ranges as recognized by the American Heart Association are:

Normal

Blood pressure numbers of less than 120/80 mm Hg are considered within the normal range. If your results fall into this category, stick with heart-healthy habits like following a balanced diet and getting regular exercise.

Elevated

Elevated blood pressure is when readings consistently range from 120-129 systolic and less than 80 mm Hg diastolic. People with elevated blood pressure are likely to develop high blood pressure unless steps are taken to control the condition.

Hypertension Stage 1

Hypertension Stage 1 is when blood pressure consistently ranges from 130-139 systolic or 80-89 mm Hg diastolic. At this stage of high blood pressure, doctors are likely to prescribe lifestyle changes and may consider adding blood pressure medication based on your risk of atherosclerotic cardiovascular disease (ASCVD), such as heart attack or stroke.

Hypertension Stage 2

Hypertension Stage 2 is when blood pressure consistently ranges at 140/90 mm Hg or higher. At this stage of high blood pressure, doctors are likely to prescribe a combination of blood pressure medications and lifestyle changes.

Hypertensive crisis

This stage of high blood pressure requires medical attention. If your blood pressure readings suddenly exceed 180/120 mm Hg, wait five minutes and then test your blood pressure again. If your readings are still unusually high, contact your doctor immediately. You could be experiencing a hypertensive crisis.

If your blood pressure is higher than 180/120 mm Hg and you are experiencing signs of possible organ damage such as chest pain, shortness of breath, back pain, numbness/weakness, change in vision or difficulty speaking, do not wait to see if your pressure comes down on its own. Call 911.

Blood Pressure Log

Month: 6-21-22

Week Starting:_____

Time		Blood Pressure		Heart Rate (Pulse Per Minute)	Notes e.g. Medication Change, Activities.
		Systolic (Upper #)	Diastolic (Lower #)		
Monday	a.m.				
	a.m.				
	3:?? p.m.	155	72	97	
	8 p.m.	130	76	83	
Tuesday	7 a.m.	134	71	93	
	a.m.				
	7 p.m.	140	74	110	
	p.m.				
Wednesday	a.m.				
	a.m.				
	p.m.				
	p.m.				
Thursday	a.m.				
	a.m.				
	p.m.				
	p.m.				
Friday	a.m.				
	a.m.				
	p.m.				
	p.m.				
Saturday	a.m.				
	a.m.				
	p.m.				
	p.m.				
Sunday	a.m.				
	a.m.				
	p.m.				
	p.m.				

Blood Pressure Log

Month:_____   Week Starting:_____

Time		Blood Pressure		Heart Rate (Pulse Per Minute)	Notes e.g. Medication Change, Activities.
		Systolic (Upper #)	Diastolic (Lower #)		
Monday	a.m.				
	a.m.				
	p.m.				
	p.m.				
Tuesday	a.m.				
	a.m.				
	p.m.				
	p.m.				
Wednesday	a.m.				
	a.m.				
	p.m.				
	p.m.				
Thursday	a.m.				
	a.m.				
	p.m.				
	p.m.				
Friday	a.m.				
	a.m.				
	p.m.				
	p.m.				
Saturday	a.m.				
	a.m.				
	p.m.				
	p.m.				
Sunday	a.m.				
	a.m.				
	p.m.				
	p.m.				

Blood Pressure Log

Month:_____   Week Starting:_____

Time	Blood Pressure		Heart Rate (Pulse Per Minute)	Notes e.g. Medication Change, Activities.
	Systolic (Upper #)	Diastolic (Lower #)		
Monday a.m.				
a.m.				
p.m.				
p.m.				
Tuesday a.m.				
a.m.				
p.m.				
p.m.				
Wednesday a.m.				
a.m.				
p.m.				
p.m.				
Thursday a.m.				
a.m.				
p.m.				
p.m.				
Friday a.m.				
a.m.				
p.m.				
p.m.				
Saturday a.m.				
a.m.				
p.m.				
p.m.				
Sunday a.m.				
a.m.				
p.m.				
p.m.				

Blood Pressure Log

Month:_____   Week Starting:_____

Time	Blood Pressure		Heart Rate (Pulse Per Minute)	Notes e.g. Medication Change, Activities.
	Systolic (Upper #)	Diastolic (Lower #)		
Monday a.m.				
a.m.				
p.m.				
p.m.				
Tuesday a.m.				
a.m.				
p.m.				
p.m.				
Wednesday a.m.				
a.m.				
p.m.				
p.m.				
Thursday a.m.				
a.m.				
p.m.				
p.m.				
Friday a.m.				
a.m.				
p.m.				
p.m.				
Saturday a.m.				
a.m.				
p.m.				
p.m.				
Sunday a.m.				
a.m.				
p.m.				
p.m.				

Blood Pressure Log

Month:_____   Week Starting:_____

Time		Blood Pressure		Heart Rate (Pulse Per Minute)	Notes e.g. Medication Change, Activities.
		Systolic (Upper #)	Diastolic (Lower #)		
Monday	a.m.				
	a.m.				
	p.m.				
	p.m.				
Tuesday	a.m.				
	a.m.				
	p.m.				
	p.m.				
Wednesday	a.m.				
	a.m.				
	p.m.				
	p.m.				
Thursday	a.m.				
	a.m.				
	p.m.				
	p.m.				
Friday	a.m.				
	a.m.				
	p.m.				
	p.m.				
Saturday	a.m.				
	a.m.				
	p.m.				
	p.m.				
Sunday	a.m.				
	a.m.				
	p.m.				
	p.m.				

Blood Pressure Log

Month:_____   Week Starting:_____

Time	Blood Pressure		Heart Rate (Pulse Per Minute)	Notes e.g. Medication Change, Activities.
	Systolic (Upper #)	Diastolic (Lower #)		
Monday a.m.				
a.m.				
p.m.				
p.m.				
Tuesday a.m.				
a.m.				
p.m.				
p.m.				
Wednesday a.m.				
a.m.				
p.m.				
p.m.				
Thursday a.m.				
a.m.				
p.m.				
p.m.				
Friday a.m.				
a.m.				
p.m.				
p.m.				
Saturday a.m.				
a.m.				
p.m.				
p.m.				
Sunday a.m.				
a.m.				
p.m.				
p.m.				

Blood Pressure Log

Month:_____   Week Starting:_____

Time		Blood Pressure		Heart Rate (Pulse Per Minute)	Notes e.g. Medication Change, Activities.
		Systolic (Upper #)	Diastolic (Lower #)		
Monday	a.m.				
	a.m.				
	p.m.				
	p.m.				
Tuesday	a.m.				
	a.m.				
	p.m.				
	p.m.				
Wednesday	a.m.				
	a.m.				
	p.m.				
	p.m.				
Thursday	a.m.				
	a.m.				
	p.m.				
	p.m.				
Friday	a.m.				
	a.m.				
	p.m.				
	p.m.				
Saturday	a.m.				
	a.m.				
	p.m.				
	p.m.				
Sunday	a.m.				
	a.m.				
	p.m.				
	p.m.				

Blood Pressure Log

Month:_____   Week Starting:_____

Time	Blood Pressure		Heart Rate (Pulse Per Minute)	Notes e.g. Medication Change, Activities.
	Systolic (Upper #)	Diastolic (Lower #)		
Monday a.m.				
a.m.				
p.m.				
p.m.				
Tuesday a.m.				
a.m.				
p.m.				
p.m.				
Wednesday a.m.				
a.m.				
p.m.				
p.m.				
Thursday a.m.				
a.m.				
p.m.				
p.m.				
Friday a.m.				
a.m.				
p.m.				
p.m.				
Saturday a.m.				
a.m.				
p.m.				
p.m.				
Sunday a.m.				
a.m.				
p.m.				
p.m.				

Blood Pressure Log

Month:_____   Week Starting:_____

Time		Blood Pressure		Heart Rate (Pulse Per Minute)	Notes e.g. Medication Change, Activities.
		Systolic (Upper #)	Diastolic (Lower #)		
Monday	a.m.				
	a.m.				
	p.m.				
	p.m.				
Tuesday	a.m.				
	a.m.				
	p.m.				
	p.m.				
Wednesday	a.m.				
	a.m.				
	p.m.				
	p.m.				
Thursday	a.m.				
	a.m.				
	p.m.				
	p.m.				
Friday	a.m.				
	a.m.				
	p.m.				
	p.m.				
Saturday	a.m.				
	a.m.				
	p.m.				
	p.m.				
Sunday	a.m.				
	a.m.				
	p.m.				
	p.m.				

Blood Pressure Log

Month:_____   Week Starting:_____

Time	Blood Pressure		Heart Rate (Pulse Per Minute)	Notes e.g. Medication Change, Activities.
	Systolic (Upper #)	Diastolic (Lower #)		
Monday a.m.				
a.m.				
p.m.				
p.m.				
Tuesday a.m.				
a.m.				
p.m.				
p.m.				
Wednesday a.m.				
a.m.				
p.m.				
p.m.				
Thursday a.m.				
a.m.				
p.m.				
p.m.				
Friday a.m.				
a.m.				
p.m.				
p.m.				
Saturday a.m.				
a.m.				
p.m.				
p.m.				
Sunday a.m.				
a.m.				
p.m.				
p.m.				

Blood Pressure Log

Month:_____   Week Starting:_____

Time		Blood Pressure		Heart Rate (Pulse Per Minute)	Notes e.g. Medication Change, Activities.
		Systolic (Upper #)	Diastolic (Lower #)		
Monday	a.m.				
	a.m.				
	p.m.				
	p.m.				
Tuesday	a.m.				
	a.m.				
	p.m.				
	p.m.				
Wednesday	a.m.				
	a.m.				
	p.m.				
	p.m.				
Thursday	a.m.				
	a.m.				
	p.m.				
	p.m.				
Friday	a.m.				
	a.m.				
	p.m.				
	p.m.				
Saturday	a.m.				
	a.m.				
	p.m.				
	p.m.				
Sunday	a.m.				
	a.m.				
	p.m.				
	p.m.				

Blood Pressure Log

Month:_____   Week Starting:_____

Time		Blood Pressure		Heart Rate (Pulse Per Minute)	Notes e.g. Medication Change, Activities.
		Systolic (Upper #)	Diastolic (Lower #)		
Monday	a.m.				
	a.m.				
	p.m.				
	p.m.				
Tuesday	a.m.				
	a.m.				
	p.m.				
	p.m.				
Wednesday	a.m.				
	a.m.				
	p.m.				
	p.m.				
Thursday	a.m.				
	a.m.				
	p.m.				
	p.m.				
Friday	a.m.				
	a.m.				
	p.m.				
	p.m.				
Saturday	a.m.				
	a.m.				
	p.m.				
	p.m.				
Sunday	a.m.				
	a.m.				
	p.m.				
	p.m.				

Blood Pressure Log

Month:_____   Week Starting:_____

Time	Blood Pressure		Heart Rate (Pulse Per Minute)	Notes e.g. Medication Change, Activities.
	Systolic (Upper #)	Diastolic (Lower #)		
Monday a.m.				
a.m.				
p.m.				
p.m.				
Tuesday a.m.				
a.m.				
p.m.				
p.m.				
Wednesday a.m.				
a.m.				
p.m.				
p.m.				
Thursday a.m.				
a.m.				
p.m.				
p.m.				
Friday a.m.				
a.m.				
p.m.				
p.m.				
Saturday a.m.				
a.m.				
p.m.				
p.m.				
Sunday a.m.				
a.m.				
p.m.				
p.m.				

Blood Pressure Log

Month:_____   Week Starting:_____

Time		Blood Pressure		Heart Rate (Pulse Per Minute)	Notes e.g. Medication Change, Activities.
		Systolic (Upper #)	Diastolic (Lower #)		
Monday	a.m.				
	a.m.				
	p.m.				
	p.m.				
Tuesday	a.m.				
	a.m.				
	p.m.				
	p.m.				
Wednesday	a.m.				
	a.m.				
	p.m.				
	p.m.				
Thursday	a.m.				
	a.m.				
	p.m.				
	p.m.				
Friday	a.m.				
	a.m.				
	p.m.				
	p.m.				
Saturday	a.m.				
	a.m.				
	p.m.				
	p.m.				
Sunday	a.m.				
	a.m.				
	p.m.				
	p.m.				

Blood Pressure Log

Month:_____   Week Starting:_____

Time		Blood Pressure		Heart Rate (Pulse Per Minute)	Notes e.g. Medication Change, Activities.
		Systolic (Upper #)	Diastolic (Lower #)		
Monday	a.m.				
	a.m.				
	p.m.				
	p.m.				
Tuesday	a.m.				
	a.m.				
	p.m.				
	p.m.				
Wednesday	a.m.				
	a.m.				
	p.m.				
	p.m.				
Thursday	a.m.				
	a.m.				
	p.m.				
	p.m.				
Friday	a.m.				
	a.m.				
	p.m.				
	p.m.				
Saturday	a.m.				
	a.m.				
	p.m.				
	p.m.				
Sunday	a.m.				
	a.m.				
	p.m.				
	p.m.				

Blood Pressure Log

Month:_____   Week Starting:_____

Time	Blood Pressure		Heart Rate (Pulse Per Minute)	Notes e.g. Medication Change, Activities.
	Systolic (Upper #)	Diastolic (Lower #)		
Monday a.m.				
a.m.				
p.m.				
p.m.				
Tuesday a.m.				
a.m.				
p.m.				
p.m.				
Wednesday a.m.				
a.m.				
p.m.				
p.m.				
Thursday a.m.				
a.m.				
p.m.				
p.m.				
Friday a.m.				
a.m.				
p.m.				
p.m.				
Saturday a.m.				
a.m.				
p.m.				
p.m.				
Sunday a.m.				
a.m.				
p.m.				
p.m.				

Blood Pressure Log

Month:_____   Week Starting:_____

Time		Blood Pressure		Heart Rate (Pulse Per Minute)	Notes e.g. Medication Change, Activities.
		Systolic (Upper #)	Diastolic (Lower #)		
Monday	a.m.				
	a.m.				
	p.m.				
	p.m.				
Tuesday	a.m.				
	a.m.				
	p.m.				
	p.m.				
Wednesday	a.m.				
	a.m.				
	p.m.				
	p.m.				
Thursday	a.m.				
	a.m.				
	p.m.				
	p.m.				
Friday	a.m.				
	a.m.				
	p.m.				
	p.m.				
Saturday	a.m.				
	a.m.				
	p.m.				
	p.m.				
Sunday	a.m.				
	a.m.				
	p.m.				
	p.m.				

Blood Pressure Log

Month:_____   Week Starting:_____

Time		Blood Pressure		Heart Rate (Pulse Per Minute)	Notes e.g. Medication Change, Activities.
		Systolic (Upper #)	Diastolic (Lower #)		
Monday	a.m.				
	a.m.				
	p.m.				
	p.m.				
Tuesday	a.m.				
	a.m.				
	p.m.				
	p.m.				
Wednesday	a.m.				
	a.m.				
	p.m.				
	p.m.				
Thursday	a.m.				
	a.m.				
	p.m.				
	p.m.				
Friday	a.m.				
	a.m.				
	p.m.				
	p.m.				
Saturday	a.m.				
	a.m.				
	p.m.				
	p.m.				
Sunday	a.m.				
	a.m.				
	p.m.				
	p.m.				

Blood Pressure Log

Month:_____   Week Starting:_____

Time		Blood Pressure		Heart Rate (Pulse Per Minute)	Notes e.g. Medication Change, Activities.
		Systolic (Upper #)	Diastolic (Lower #)		
Monday	a.m.				
	a.m.				
	p.m.				
	p.m.				
Tuesday	a.m.				
	a.m.				
	p.m.				
	p.m.				
Wednesday	a.m.				
	a.m.				
	p.m.				
	p.m.				
Thursday	a.m.				
	a.m.				
	p.m.				
	p.m.				
Friday	a.m.				
	a.m.				
	p.m.				
	p.m.				
Saturday	a.m.				
	a.m.				
	p.m.				
	p.m.				
Sunday	a.m.				
	a.m.				
	p.m.				
	p.m.				

Blood Pressure Log

Month:_____   Week Starting:_____

Time		Blood Pressure		Heart Rate (Pulse Per Minute)	Notes e.g. Medication Change, Activities.
		Systolic (Upper #)	Diastolic (Lower #)		
Monday	a.m.				
	a.m.				
	p.m.				
	p.m.				
Tuesday	a.m.				
	a.m.				
	p.m.				
	p.m.				
Wednesday	a.m.				
	a.m.				
	p.m.				
	p.m.				
Thursday	a.m.				
	a.m.				
	p.m.				
	p.m.				
Friday	a.m.				
	a.m.				
	p.m.				
	p.m.				
Saturday	a.m.				
	a.m.				
	p.m.				
	p.m.				
Sunday	a.m.				
	a.m.				
	p.m.				
	p.m.				

Blood Pressure Log

Month:_____   Week Starting:_____

Time	Blood Pressure		Heart Rate (Pulse Per Minute)	Notes e.g. Medication Change, Activities.
	Systolic (Upper #)	Diastolic (Lower #)		
Monday a.m.				
a.m.				
p.m.				
p.m.				
Tuesday a.m.				
a.m.				
p.m.				
p.m.				
Wednesday a.m.				
a.m.				
p.m.				
p.m.				
Thursday a.m.				
a.m.				
p.m.				
p.m.				
Friday a.m.				
a.m.				
p.m.				
p.m.				
Saturday a.m.				
a.m.				
p.m.				
p.m.				
Sunday a.m.				
a.m.				
p.m.				
p.m.				

Blood Pressure Log

Month:_____   Week Starting:_____

Time	Blood Pressure		Heart Rate (Pulse Per Minute)	Notes e.g. Medication Change, Activities.
	Systolic (Upper #)	Diastolic (Lower #)		
Monday a.m.				
a.m.				
p.m.				
p.m.				
Tuesday a.m.				
a.m.				
p.m.				
p.m.				
Wednesday a.m.				
a.m.				
p.m.				
p.m.				
Thursday a.m.				
a.m.				
p.m.				
p.m.				
Friday a.m.				
a.m.				
p.m.				
p.m.				
Saturday a.m.				
a.m.				
p.m.				
p.m.				
Sunday a.m.				
a.m.				
p.m.				
p.m.				

Blood Pressure Log

Month:_____   Week Starting:_____

Time		Blood Pressure		Heart Rate (Pulse Per Minute)	Notes e.g. Medication Change, Activities.
		Systolic (Upper #)	Diastolic (Lower #)		
Monday	a.m.				
	a.m.				
	p.m.				
	p.m.				
Tuesday	a.m.				
	a.m.				
	p.m.				
	p.m.				
Wednesday	a.m.				
	a.m.				
	p.m.				
	p.m.				
Thursday	a.m.				
	a.m.				
	p.m.				
	p.m.				
Friday	a.m.				
	a.m.				
	p.m.				
	p.m.				
Saturday	a.m.				
	a.m.				
	p.m.				
	p.m.				
Sunday	a.m.				
	a.m.				
	p.m.				
	p.m.				

Blood Pressure Log

Month:_____   Week Starting:_____

Time		Blood Pressure		Heart Rate (Pulse Per Minute)	Notes e.g. Medication Change, Activities.
		Systolic (Upper #)	Diastolic (Lower #)		
Monday	a.m.				
	a.m.				
	p.m.				
	p.m.				
Tuesday	a.m.				
	a.m.				
	p.m.				
	p.m.				
Wednesday	a.m.				
	a.m.				
	p.m.				
	p.m.				
Thursday	a.m.				
	a.m.				
	p.m.				
	p.m.				
Friday	a.m.				
	a.m.				
	p.m.				
	p.m.				
Saturday	a.m.				
	a.m.				
	p.m.				
	p.m.				
Sunday	a.m.				
	a.m.				
	p.m.				
	p.m.				

Blood Pressure Log

Month:_____   Week Starting:_____

Time	Blood Pressure		Heart Rate (Pulse Per Minute)	Notes e.g. Medication Change, Activities.
	Systolic (Upper #)	Diastolic (Lower #)		
Monday a.m.				
a.m.				
p.m.				
p.m.				
Tuesday a.m.				
a.m.				
p.m.				
p.m.				
Wednesday a.m.				
a.m.				
p.m.				
p.m.				
Thursday a.m.				
a.m.				
p.m.				
p.m.				
Friday a.m.				
a.m.				
p.m.				
p.m.				
Saturday a.m.				
a.m.				
p.m.				
p.m.				
Sunday a.m.				
a.m.				
p.m.				
p.m.				

Blood Pressure Log

Month:_____   Week Starting:_____

Time		Blood Pressure		Heart Rate (Pulse Per Minute)	Notes e.g. Medication Change, Activities.
		Systolic (Upper #)	Diastolic (Lower #)		
Monday	a.m.				
	a.m.				
	p.m.				
	p.m.				
Tuesday	a.m.				
	a.m.				
	p.m.				
	p.m.				
Wednesday	a.m.				
	a.m.				
	p.m.				
	p.m.				
Thursday	a.m.				
	a.m.				
	p.m.				
	p.m.				
Friday	a.m.				
	a.m.				
	p.m.				
	p.m.				
Saturday	a.m.				
	a.m.				
	p.m.				
	p.m.				
Sunday	a.m.				
	a.m.				
	p.m.				
	p.m.				

Blood Pressure Log

Month:_____   Week Starting:_____

Time		Blood Pressure		Heart Rate (Pulse Per Minute)	Notes e.g. Medication Change, Activities.
		Systolic (Upper #)	Diastolic (Lower #)		
Monday	a.m.				
	a.m.				
	p.m.				
	p.m.				
Tuesday	a.m.				
	a.m.				
	p.m.				
	p.m.				
Wednesday	a.m.				
	a.m.				
	p.m.				
	p.m.				
Thursday	a.m.				
	a.m.				
	p.m.				
	p.m.				
Friday	a.m.				
	a.m.				
	p.m.				
	p.m.				
Saturday	a.m.				
	a.m.				
	p.m.				
	p.m.				
Sunday	a.m.				
	a.m.				
	p.m.				
	p.m.				

Blood Pressure Log

Month:_____   Week Starting:_____

Time	Blood Pressure		Heart Rate (Pulse Per Minute)	Notes e.g. Medication Change, Activities.
	Systolic (Upper #)	Diastolic (Lower #)		
Monday a.m.				
a.m.				
p.m.				
p.m.				
Tuesday a.m.				
a.m.				
p.m.				
p.m.				
Wednesday a.m.				
a.m.				
p.m.				
p.m.				
Thursday a.m.				
a.m.				
p.m.				
p.m.				
Friday a.m.				
a.m.				
p.m.				
p.m.				
Saturday a.m.				
a.m.				
p.m.				
p.m.				
Sunday a.m.				
a.m.				
p.m.				
p.m.				

Blood Pressure Log

Month:_____   Week Starting:_____

Time		Blood Pressure		Heart Rate (Pulse Per Minute)	Notes e.g. Medication Change, Activities.
		Systolic (Upper #)	Diastolic (Lower #)		
Monday	a.m.				
	a.m.				
	p.m.				
	p.m.				
Tuesday	a.m.				
	a.m.				
	p.m.				
	p.m.				
Wednesday	a.m.				
	a.m.				
	p.m.				
	p.m.				
Thursday	a.m.				
	a.m.				
	p.m.				
	p.m.				
Friday	a.m.				
	a.m.				
	p.m.				
	p.m.				
Saturday	a.m.				
	a.m.				
	p.m.				
	p.m.				
Sunday	a.m.				
	a.m.				
	p.m.				
	p.m.				

Blood Pressure Log

Month:_____   Week Starting:_____

Time		Blood Pressure		Heart Rate (Pulse Per Minute)	Notes e.g. Medication Change, Activities.
		Systolic (Upper #)	Diastolic (Lower #)		
Monday	a.m.				
	a.m.				
	p.m.				
	p.m.				
Tuesday	a.m.				
	a.m.				
	p.m.				
	p.m.				
Wednesday	a.m.				
	a.m.				
	p.m.				
	p.m.				
Thursday	a.m.				
	a.m.				
	p.m.				
	p.m.				
Friday	a.m.				
	a.m.				
	p.m.				
	p.m.				
Saturday	a.m.				
	a.m.				
	p.m.				
	p.m.				
Sunday	a.m.				
	a.m.				
	p.m.				
	p.m.				

Blood Pressure Log

Month:_____   Week Starting:_____

Time		Blood Pressure		Heart Rate (Pulse Per Minute)	Notes e.g. Medication Change, Activities.
		Systolic (Upper #)	Diastolic (Lower #)		
Monday	a.m.				
	a.m.				
	p.m.				
	p.m.				
Tuesday	a.m.				
	a.m.				
	p.m.				
	p.m.				
Wednesday	a.m.				
	a.m.				
	p.m.				
	p.m.				
Thursday	a.m.				
	a.m.				
	p.m.				
	p.m.				
Friday	a.m.				
	a.m.				
	p.m.				
	p.m.				
Saturday	a.m.				
	a.m.				
	p.m.				
	p.m.				
Sunday	a.m.				
	a.m.				
	p.m.				
	p.m.				

Blood Pressure Log

Month:_____   Week Starting:_____

Time		Blood Pressure		Heart Rate (Pulse Per Minute)	Notes e.g. Medication Change, Activities.
		Systolic (Upper #)	Diastolic (Lower #)		
Monday	a.m.				
	a.m.				
	p.m.				
	p.m.				
Tuesday	a.m.				
	a.m.				
	p.m.				
	p.m.				
Wednesday	a.m.				
	a.m.				
	p.m.				
	p.m.				
Thursday	a.m.				
	a.m.				
	p.m.				
	p.m.				
Friday	a.m.				
	a.m.				
	p.m.				
	p.m.				
Saturday	a.m.				
	a.m.				
	p.m.				
	p.m.				
Sunday	a.m.				
	a.m.				
	p.m.				
	p.m.				

Blood Pressure Log

Month:_____   Week Starting:_____

Time	Blood Pressure		Heart Rate (Pulse Per Minute)	Notes e.g. Medication Change, Activities.
	Systolic (Upper #)	Diastolic (Lower #)		
Monday a.m.				
a.m.				
p.m.				
p.m.				
Tuesday a.m.				
a.m.				
p.m.				
p.m.				
Wednesday a.m.				
a.m.				
p.m.				
p.m.				
Thursday a.m.				
a.m.				
p.m.				
p.m.				
Friday a.m.				
a.m.				
p.m.				
p.m.				
Saturday a.m.				
a.m.				
p.m.				
p.m.				
Sunday a.m.				
a.m.				
p.m.				
p.m.				

Blood Pressure Log

Month:_____   Week Starting:_____

Time	Blood Pressure		Heart Rate (Pulse Per Minute)	Notes e.g. Medication Change, Activities.
	Systolic (Upper #)	Diastolic (Lower #)		
Monday a.m.				
a.m.				
p.m.				
p.m.				
Tuesday a.m.				
a.m.				
p.m.				
p.m.				
Wednesday a.m.				
a.m.				
p.m.				
p.m.				
Thursday a.m.				
a.m.				
p.m.				
p.m.				
Friday a.m.				
a.m.				
p.m.				
p.m.				
Saturday a.m.				
a.m.				
p.m.				
p.m.				
Sunday a.m.				
a.m.				
p.m.				
p.m.				

Blood Pressure Log

Month:_____   Week Starting:_____

Time		Blood Pressure		Heart Rate (Pulse Per Minute)	Notes e.g. Medication Change, Activities.
		Systolic (Upper #)	Diastolic (Lower #)		
Monday	a.m.				
	a.m.				
	p.m.				
	p.m.				
Tuesday	a.m.				
	a.m.				
	p.m.				
	p.m.				
Wednesday	a.m.				
	a.m.				
	p.m.				
	p.m.				
Thursday	a.m.				
	a.m.				
	p.m.				
	p.m.				
Friday	a.m.				
	a.m.				
	p.m.				
	p.m.				
Saturday	a.m.				
	a.m.				
	p.m.				
	p.m.				
Sunday	a.m.				
	a.m.				
	p.m.				
	p.m.				

Blood Pressure Log

Month:_____   Week Starting:_____

Time		Blood Pressure		Heart Rate (Pulse Per Minute)	Notes e.g. Medication Change, Activities.
		Systolic (Upper #)	Diastolic (Lower #)		
Monday	a.m.				
	a.m.				
	p.m.				
	p.m.				
Tuesday	a.m.				
	a.m.				
	p.m.				
	p.m.				
Wednesday	a.m.				
	a.m.				
	p.m.				
	p.m.				
Thursday	a.m.				
	a.m.				
	p.m.				
	p.m.				
Friday	a.m.				
	a.m.				
	p.m.				
	p.m.				
Saturday	a.m.				
	a.m.				
	p.m.				
	p.m.				
Sunday	a.m.				
	a.m.				
	p.m.				
	p.m.				

Blood Pressure Log

Month:_____   Week Starting:_____

Time	Blood Pressure		Heart Rate (Pulse Per Minute)	Notes e.g. Medication Change, Activities.
	Systolic (Upper #)	Diastolic (Lower #)		
Monday a.m.				
a.m.				
p.m.				
p.m.				
Tuesday a.m.				
a.m.				
p.m.				
p.m.				
Wednesday a.m.				
a.m.				
p.m.				
p.m.				
Thursday a.m.				
a.m.				
p.m.				
p.m.				
Friday a.m.				
a.m.				
p.m.				
p.m.				
Saturday a.m.				
a.m.				
p.m.				
p.m.				
Sunday a.m.				
a.m.				
p.m.				
p.m.				

Blood Pressure Log

Month:_____   Week Starting:_____

Time		Blood Pressure		Heart Rate (Pulse Per Minute)	Notes e.g. Medication Change, Activities.
		Systolic (Upper #)	Diastolic (Lower #)		
Monday	a.m.				
	a.m.				
	p.m.				
	p.m.				
Tuesday	a.m.				
	a.m.				
	p.m.				
	p.m.				
Wednesday	a.m.				
	a.m.				
	p.m.				
	p.m.				
Thursday	a.m.				
	a.m.				
	p.m.				
	p.m.				
Friday	a.m.				
	a.m.				
	p.m.				
	p.m.				
Saturday	a.m.				
	a.m.				
	p.m.				
	p.m.				
Sunday	a.m.				
	a.m.				
	p.m.				
	p.m.				

Blood Pressure Log

Month:_____   Week Starting:_____

Time		Blood Pressure		Heart Rate (Pulse Per Minute)	Notes e.g. Medication Change, Activities.
		Systolic (Upper #)	Diastolic (Lower #)		
Monday	a.m.				
	a.m.				
	p.m.				
	p.m.				
Tuesday	a.m.				
	a.m.				
	p.m.				
	p.m.				
Wednesday	a.m.				
	a.m.				
	p.m.				
	p.m.				
Thursday	a.m.				
	a.m.				
	p.m.				
	p.m.				
Friday	a.m.				
	a.m.				
	p.m.				
	p.m.				
Saturday	a.m.				
	a.m.				
	p.m.				
	p.m.				
Sunday	a.m.				
	a.m.				
	p.m.				
	p.m.				

Blood Pressure Log

Month:_____   Week Starting:_____

Time		Blood Pressure		Heart Rate (Pulse Per Minute)	Notes e.g. Medication Change, Activities.
		Systolic (Upper #)	Diastolic (Lower #)		
Monday	a.m.				
	a.m.				
	p.m.				
	p.m.				
Tuesday	a.m.				
	a.m.				
	p.m.				
	p.m.				
Wednesday	a.m.				
	a.m.				
	p.m.				
	p.m.				
Thursday	a.m.				
	a.m.				
	p.m.				
	p.m.				
Friday	a.m.				
	a.m.				
	p.m.				
	p.m.				
Saturday	a.m.				
	a.m.				
	p.m.				
	p.m.				
Sunday	a.m.				
	a.m.				
	p.m.				
	p.m.				

Blood Pressure Log

Month:_____   Week Starting:_____

Time		Blood Pressure		Heart Rate (Pulse Per Minute)	Notes e.g. Medication Change, Activities.
		Systolic (Upper #)	Diastolic (Lower #)		
Monday	a.m.				
	a.m.				
	p.m.				
	p.m.				
Tuesday	a.m.				
	a.m.				
	p.m.				
	p.m.				
Wednesday	a.m.				
	a.m.				
	p.m.				
	p.m.				
Thursday	a.m.				
	a.m.				
	p.m.				
	p.m.				
Friday	a.m.				
	a.m.				
	p.m.				
	p.m.				
Saturday	a.m.				
	a.m.				
	p.m.				
	p.m.				
Sunday	a.m.				
	a.m.				
	p.m.				
	p.m.				

Blood Pressure Log

Month:_____   Week Starting:_____

Time	Blood Pressure		Heart Rate (Pulse Per Minute)	Notes e.g. Medication Change, Activities.
	Systolic (Upper #)	Diastolic (Lower #)		
Monday a.m.				
a.m.				
p.m.				
p.m.				
Tuesday a.m.				
a.m.				
p.m.				
p.m.				
Wednesday a.m.				
a.m.				
p.m.				
p.m.				
Thursday a.m.				
a.m.				
p.m.				
p.m.				
Friday a.m.				
a.m.				
p.m.				
p.m.				
Saturday a.m.				
a.m.				
p.m.				
p.m.				
Sunday a.m.				
a.m.				
p.m.				
p.m.				

Blood Pressure Log

Month:_____   Week Starting:_____

Time		Blood Pressure		Heart Rate (Pulse Per Minute)	Notes e.g. Medication Change, Activities.
		Systolic (Upper #)	Diastolic (Lower #)		
Monday	a.m.				
Monday	a.m.				
Monday	p.m.				
Monday	p.m.				
Tuesday	a.m.				
Tuesday	a.m.				
Tuesday	p.m.				
Tuesday	p.m.				
Wednesday	a.m.				
Wednesday	a.m.				
Wednesday	p.m.				
Wednesday	p.m.				
Thursday	a.m.				
Thursday	a.m.				
Thursday	p.m.				
Thursday	p.m.				
Friday	a.m.				
Friday	a.m.				
Friday	p.m.				
Friday	p.m.				
Saturday	a.m.				
Saturday	a.m.				
Saturday	p.m.				
Saturday	p.m.				
Sunday	a.m.				
Sunday	a.m.				
Sunday	p.m.				
Sunday	p.m.				

Blood Pressure Log

Month:_____   Week Starting:_____

Time		Blood Pressure		Heart Rate (Pulse Per Minute)	Notes e.g. Medication Change, Activities.
		Systolic (Upper #)	Diastolic (Lower #)		
Monday	a.m.				
	a.m.				
	p.m.				
	p.m.				
Tuesday	a.m.				
	a.m.				
	p.m.				
	p.m.				
Wednesday	a.m.				
	a.m.				
	p.m.				
	p.m.				
Thursday	a.m.				
	a.m.				
	p.m.				
	p.m.				
Friday	a.m.				
	a.m.				
	p.m.				
	p.m.				
Saturday	a.m.				
	a.m.				
	p.m.				
	p.m.				
Sunday	a.m.				
	a.m.				
	p.m.				
	p.m.				

Blood Pressure Log

Month:_____   Week Starting:_____

Time	Blood Pressure		Heart Rate (Pulse Per Minute)	Notes e.g. Medication Change, Activities.
	Systolic (Upper #)	Diastolic (Lower #)		
Monday a.m.				
a.m.				
p.m.				
p.m.				
Tuesday a.m.				
a.m.				
p.m.				
p.m.				
Wednesday a.m.				
a.m.				
p.m.				
p.m.				
Thursday a.m.				
a.m.				
p.m.				
p.m.				
Friday a.m.				
a.m.				
p.m.				
p.m.				
Saturday a.m.				
a.m.				
p.m.				
p.m.				
Sunday a.m.				
a.m.				
p.m.				
p.m.				

Blood Pressure Log

Month:_____   Week Starting:_____

Time	Blood Pressure		Heart Rate (Pulse Per Minute)	Notes e.g. Medication Change, Activities.
	Systolic (Upper #)	Diastolic (Lower #)		
Monday a.m.				
a.m.				
p.m.				
p.m.				
Tuesday a.m.				
a.m.				
p.m.				
p.m.				
Wednesday a.m.				
a.m.				
p.m.				
p.m.				
Thursday a.m.				
a.m.				
p.m.				
p.m.				
Friday a.m.				
a.m.				
p.m.				
p.m.				
Saturday a.m.				
a.m.				
p.m.				
p.m.				
Sunday a.m.				
a.m.				
p.m.				
p.m.				

Blood Pressure Log

Month:_____   Week Starting:_____

Time	Blood Pressure		Heart Rate (Pulse Per Minute)	Notes e.g. Medication Change, Activities.
	Systolic (Upper #)	Diastolic (Lower #)		
Monday a.m.				
a.m.				
p.m.				
p.m.				
Tuesday a.m.				
a.m.				
p.m.				
p.m.				
Wednesday a.m.				
a.m.				
p.m.				
p.m.				
Thursday a.m.				
a.m.				
p.m.				
p.m.				
Friday a.m.				
a.m.				
p.m.				
p.m.				
Saturday a.m.				
a.m.				
p.m.				
p.m.				
Sunday a.m.				
a.m.				
p.m.				
p.m.				

Blood Pressure Log

Month:_____   Week Starting:_____

Time		Blood Pressure		Heart Rate (Pulse Per Minute)	Notes e.g. Medication Change, Activities.
		Systolic (Upper #)	Diastolic (Lower #)		
Monday	a.m.				
	a.m.				
	p.m.				
	p.m.				
Tuesday	a.m.				
	a.m.				
	p.m.				
	p.m.				
Wednesday	a.m.				
	a.m.				
	p.m.				
	p.m.				
Thursday	a.m.				
	a.m.				
	p.m.				
	p.m.				
Friday	a.m.				
	a.m.				
	p.m.				
	p.m.				
Saturday	a.m.				
	a.m.				
	p.m.				
	p.m.				
Sunday	a.m.				
	a.m.				
	p.m.				
	p.m.				

Blood Pressure Log

Month:_____   Week Starting:_____

Time		Blood Pressure		Heart Rate (Pulse Per Minute)	Notes e.g. Medication Change, Activities.
		Systolic (Upper #)	Diastolic (Lower #)		
Monday	a.m.				
	a.m.				
	p.m.				
	p.m.				
Tuesday	a.m.				
	a.m.				
	p.m.				
	p.m.				
Wednesday	a.m.				
	a.m.				
	p.m.				
	p.m.				
Thursday	a.m.				
	a.m.				
	p.m.				
	p.m.				
Friday	a.m.				
	a.m.				
	p.m.				
	p.m.				
Saturday	a.m.				
	a.m.				
	p.m.				
	p.m.				
Sunday	a.m.				
	a.m.				
	p.m.				
	p.m.				

Blood Pressure Log

Month:_____   Week Starting:_____

Time		Blood Pressure		Heart Rate (Pulse Per Minute)	Notes e.g. Medication Change, Activities.
		Systolic (Upper #)	Diastolic (Lower #)		
Monday	a.m.				
	a.m.				
	p.m.				
	p.m.				
Tuesday	a.m.				
	a.m.				
	p.m.				
	p.m.				
Wednesday	a.m.				
	a.m.				
	p.m.				
	p.m.				
Thursday	a.m.				
	a.m.				
	p.m.				
	p.m.				
Friday	a.m.				
	a.m.				
	p.m.				
	p.m.				
Saturday	a.m.				
	a.m.				
	p.m.				
	p.m.				
Sunday	a.m.				
	a.m.				
	p.m.				
	p.m.				

Blood Pressure Log

Month:_____   Week Starting:_____

Time		Blood Pressure		Heart Rate (Pulse Per Minute)	Notes e.g. Medication Change, Activities.
		Systolic (Upper #)	Diastolic (Lower #)		
Monday	a.m.				
	a.m.				
	p.m.				
	p.m.				
Tuesday	a.m.				
	a.m.				
	p.m.				
	p.m.				
Wednesday	a.m.				
	a.m.				
	p.m.				
	p.m.				
Thursday	a.m.				
	a.m.				
	p.m.				
	p.m.				
Friday	a.m.				
	a.m.				
	p.m.				
	p.m.				
Saturday	a.m.				
	a.m.				
	p.m.				
	p.m.				
Sunday	a.m.				
	a.m.				
	p.m.				
	p.m.				

Blood Pressure Log

Month:_____   Week Starting:_____

Time		Blood Pressure		Heart Rate (Pulse Per Minute)	Notes e.g. Medication Change, Activities.
		Systolic (Upper #)	Diastolic (Lower #)		
Monday	a.m.				
	a.m.				
	p.m.				
	p.m.				
Tuesday	a.m.				
	a.m.				
	p.m.				
	p.m.				
Wednesday	a.m.				
	a.m.				
	p.m.				
	p.m.				
Thursday	a.m.				
	a.m.				
	p.m.				
	p.m.				
Friday	a.m.				
	a.m.				
	p.m.				
	p.m.				
Saturday	a.m.				
	a.m.				
	p.m.				
	p.m.				
Sunday	a.m.				
	a.m.				
	p.m.				
	p.m.				

Blood Pressure Log

Month:_____   Week Starting:_____

Time	Blood Pressure		Heart Rate (Pulse Per Minute)	Notes e.g. Medication Change, Activities.
	Systolic (Upper #)	Diastolic (Lower #)		
Monday a.m.				
a.m.				
p.m.				
p.m.				
Tuesday a.m.				
a.m.				
p.m.				
p.m.				
Wednesday a.m.				
a.m.				
p.m.				
p.m.				
Thursday a.m.				
a.m.				
p.m.				
p.m.				
Friday a.m.				
a.m.				
p.m.				
p.m.				
Saturday a.m.				
a.m.				
p.m.				
p.m.				
Sunday a.m.				
a.m.				
p.m.				
p.m.				

Blood Pressure Log

Month:_____   Week Starting:_____

Time		Blood Pressure		Heart Rate (Pulse Per Minute)	Notes e.g. Medication Change, Activities.
		Systolic (Upper #)	Diastolic (Lower #)		
Monday	a.m.				
	a.m.				
	p.m.				
	p.m.				
Tuesday	a.m.				
	a.m.				
	p.m.				
	p.m.				
Wednesday	a.m.				
	a.m.				
	p.m.				
	p.m.				
Thursday	a.m.				
	a.m.				
	p.m.				
	p.m.				
Friday	a.m.				
	a.m.				
	p.m.				
	p.m.				
Saturday	a.m.				
	a.m.				
	p.m.				
	p.m.				
Sunday	a.m.				
	a.m.				
	p.m.				
	p.m.				

Blood Pressure Log

Month:_____   Week Starting:_____

Time		Blood Pressure		Heart Rate (Pulse Per Minute)	Notes e.g. Medication Change, Activities.
		Systolic (Upper #)	Diastolic (Lower #)		
Monday	a.m.				
	a.m.				
	p.m.				
	p.m.				
Tuesday	a.m.				
	a.m.				
	p.m.				
	p.m.				
Wednesday	a.m.				
	a.m.				
	p.m.				
	p.m.				
Thursday	a.m.				
	a.m.				
	p.m.				
	p.m.				
Friday	a.m.				
	a.m.				
	p.m.				
	p.m.				
Saturday	a.m.				
	a.m.				
	p.m.				
	p.m.				
Sunday	a.m.				
	a.m.				
	p.m.				
	p.m.				

Blood Pressure Log

Month:_____   Week Starting:_____

Time	Blood Pressure		Heart Rate (Pulse Per Minute)	Notes e.g. Medication Change, Activities.
	Systolic (Upper #)	Diastolic (Lower #)		
Monday a.m.				
a.m.				
p.m.				
p.m.				
Tuesday a.m.				
a.m.				
p.m.				
p.m.				
Wednesday a.m.				
a.m.				
p.m.				
p.m.				
Thursday a.m.				
a.m.				
p.m.				
p.m.				
Friday a.m.				
a.m.				
p.m.				
p.m.				
Saturday a.m.				
a.m.				
p.m.				
p.m.				
Sunday a.m.				
a.m.				
p.m.				
p.m.				

Blood Pressure Log

Month:_____   Week Starting:_____

Time		Blood Pressure		Heart Rate (Pulse Per Minute)	Notes e.g. Medication Change, Activities.
		Systolic (Upper #)	Diastolic (Lower #)		
Monday	a.m.				
	a.m.				
	p.m.				
	p.m.				
Tuesday	a.m.				
	a.m.				
	p.m.				
	p.m.				
Wednesday	a.m.				
	a.m.				
	p.m.				
	p.m.				
Thursday	a.m.				
	a.m.				
	p.m.				
	p.m.				
Friday	a.m.				
	a.m.				
	p.m.				
	p.m.				
Saturday	a.m.				
	a.m.				
	p.m.				
	p.m.				
Sunday	a.m.				
	a.m.				
	p.m.				
	p.m.				

Blood Pressure Log

Month:_____   Week Starting:_____

Time		Blood Pressure		Heart Rate (Pulse Per Minute)	Notes e.g. Medication Change, Activities.
		Systolic (Upper #)	Diastolic (Lower #)		
Monday	a.m.				
	a.m.				
	p.m.				
	p.m.				
Tuesday	a.m.				
	a.m.				
	p.m.				
	p.m.				
Wednesday	a.m.				
	a.m.				
	p.m.				
	p.m.				
Thursday	a.m.				
	a.m.				
	p.m.				
	p.m.				
Friday	a.m.				
	a.m.				
	p.m.				
	p.m.				
Saturday	a.m.				
	a.m.				
	p.m.				
	p.m.				
Sunday	a.m.				
	a.m.				
	p.m.				
	p.m.				

Blood Pressure Log

Month:_____   Week Starting:_____

Time		Blood Pressure		Heart Rate (Pulse Per Minute)	Notes e.g. Medication Change, Activities.
		Systolic (Upper #)	Diastolic (Lower #)		
Monday	a.m.				
Monday	a.m.				
Monday	p.m.				
Monday	p.m.				
Tuesday	a.m.				
Tuesday	a.m.				
Tuesday	p.m.				
Tuesday	p.m.				
Wednesday	a.m.				
Wednesday	a.m.				
Wednesday	p.m.				
Wednesday	p.m.				
Thursday	a.m.				
Thursday	a.m.				
Thursday	p.m.				
Thursday	p.m.				
Friday	a.m.				
Friday	a.m.				
Friday	p.m.				
Friday	p.m.				
Saturday	a.m.				
Saturday	a.m.				
Saturday	p.m.				
Saturday	p.m.				
Sunday	a.m.				
Sunday	a.m.				
Sunday	p.m.				
Sunday	p.m.				

Blood Pressure Log

Month:_____   Week Starting:_____

Time	Blood Pressure		Heart Rate (Pulse Per Minute)	Notes e.g. Medication Change, Activities.
	Systolic (Upper #)	Diastolic (Lower #)		
Monday a.m.				
a.m.				
p.m.				
p.m.				
Tuesday a.m.				
a.m.				
p.m.				
p.m.				
Wednesday a.m.				
a.m.				
p.m.				
p.m.				
Thursday a.m.				
a.m.				
p.m.				
p.m.				
Friday a.m.				
a.m.				
p.m.				
p.m.				
Saturday a.m.				
a.m.				
p.m.				
p.m.				
Sunday a.m.				
a.m.				
p.m.				
p.m.				

Blood Pressure Log

Month:_____   Week Starting:_____

Time		Blood Pressure		Heart Rate (Pulse Per Minute)	Notes e.g. Medication Change, Activities.
		Systolic (Upper #)	Diastolic (Lower #)		
Monday	a.m.				
	a.m.				
	p.m.				
	p.m.				
Tuesday	a.m.				
	a.m.				
	p.m.				
	p.m.				
Wednesday	a.m.				
	a.m.				
	p.m.				
	p.m.				
Thursday	a.m.				
	a.m.				
	p.m.				
	p.m.				
Friday	a.m.				
	a.m.				
	p.m.				
	p.m.				
Saturday	a.m.				
	a.m.				
	p.m.				
	p.m.				
Sunday	a.m.				
	a.m.				
	p.m.				
	p.m.				

Blood Pressure Log

Month:_____   Week Starting:_____

Time	Blood Pressure		Heart Rate (Pulse Per Minute)	Notes e.g. Medication Change, Activities.
	Systolic (Upper #)	Diastolic (Lower #)		
Monday a.m.				
a.m.				
p.m.				
p.m.				
Tuesday a.m.				
a.m.				
p.m.				
p.m.				
Wednesday a.m.				
a.m.				
p.m.				
p.m.				
Thursday a.m.				
a.m.				
p.m.				
p.m.				
Friday a.m.				
a.m.				
p.m.				
p.m.				
Saturday a.m.				
a.m.				
p.m.				
p.m.				
Sunday a.m.				
a.m.				
p.m.				
p.m.				

Blood Pressure Log

Month:_____   Week Starting:_____

Time		Blood Pressure		Heart Rate (Pulse Per Minute)	Notes e.g. Medication Change, Activities.
		Systolic (Upper #)	Diastolic (Lower #)		
Monday	a.m.				
	a.m.				
	p.m.				
	p.m.				
Tuesday	a.m.				
	a.m.				
	p.m.				
	p.m.				
Wednesday	a.m.				
	a.m.				
	p.m.				
	p.m.				
Thursday	a.m.				
	a.m.				
	p.m.				
	p.m.				
Friday	a.m.				
	a.m.				
	p.m.				
	p.m.				
Saturday	a.m.				
	a.m.				
	p.m.				
	p.m.				
Sunday	a.m.				
	a.m.				
	p.m.				
	p.m.				

Blood Pressure Log

Month:_____   Week Starting:_____

Time	Blood Pressure		Heart Rate (Pulse Per Minute)	Notes e.g. Medication Change, Activities.
	Systolic (Upper #)	Diastolic (Lower #)		
Monday a.m.				
a.m.				
p.m.				
p.m.				
Tuesday a.m.				
a.m.				
p.m.				
p.m.				
Wednesday a.m.				
a.m.				
p.m.				
p.m.				
Thursday a.m.				
a.m.				
p.m.				
p.m.				
Friday a.m.				
a.m.				
p.m.				
p.m.				
Saturday a.m.				
a.m.				
p.m.				
p.m.				
Sunday a.m.				
a.m.				
p.m.				
p.m.				

Blood Pressure Log

Month:_____   Week Starting:_____

Time		Blood Pressure		Heart Rate (Pulse Per Minute)	Notes e.g. Medication Change, Activities.
		Systolic (Upper #)	Diastolic (Lower #)		
Monday	a.m.				
	a.m.				
	p.m.				
	p.m.				
Tuesday	a.m.				
	a.m.				
	p.m.				
	p.m.				
Wednesday	a.m.				
	a.m.				
	p.m.				
	p.m.				
Thursday	a.m.				
	a.m.				
	p.m.				
	p.m.				
Friday	a.m.				
	a.m.				
	p.m.				
	p.m.				
Saturday	a.m.				
	a.m.				
	p.m.				
	p.m.				
Sunday	a.m.				
	a.m.				
	p.m.				
	p.m.				

Blood Pressure Log

Month:_____   Week Starting:_____

Time	Blood Pressure		Heart Rate (Pulse Per Minute)	Notes e.g. Medication Change, Activities.
	Systolic (Upper #)	Diastolic (Lower #)		
Monday a.m.				
a.m.				
p.m.				
p.m.				
Tuesday a.m.				
a.m.				
p.m.				
p.m.				
Wednesday a.m.				
a.m.				
p.m.				
p.m.				
Thursday a.m.				
a.m.				
p.m.				
p.m.				
Friday a.m.				
a.m.				
p.m.				
p.m.				
Saturday a.m.				
a.m.				
p.m.				
p.m.				
Sunday a.m.				
a.m.				
p.m.				
p.m.				

Blood Pressure Log

Month:_____   Week Starting:_____

Time	Blood Pressure		Heart Rate (Pulse Per Minute)	Notes e.g. Medication Change, Activities.
	Systolic (Upper #)	Diastolic (Lower #)		
Monday a.m.				
a.m.				
p.m.				
p.m.				
Tuesday a.m.				
a.m.				
p.m.				
p.m.				
Wednesday a.m.				
a.m.				
p.m.				
p.m.				
Thursday a.m.				
a.m.				
p.m.				
p.m.				
Friday a.m.				
a.m.				
p.m.				
p.m.				
Saturday a.m.				
a.m.				
p.m.				
p.m.				
Sunday a.m.				
a.m.				
p.m.				
p.m.				

Blood Pressure Log

Month:_____   Week Starting:_____

Time		Blood Pressure		Heart Rate (Pulse Per Minute)	Notes e.g. Medication Change, Activities.
		Systolic (Upper #)	Diastolic (Lower #)		
Monday	a.m.				
	a.m.				
	p.m.				
	p.m.				
Tuesday	a.m.				
	a.m.				
	p.m.				
	p.m.				
Wednesday	a.m.				
	a.m.				
	p.m.				
	p.m.				
Thursday	a.m.				
	a.m.				
	p.m.				
	p.m.				
Friday	a.m.				
	a.m.				
	p.m.				
	p.m.				
Saturday	a.m.				
	a.m.				
	p.m.				
	p.m.				
Sunday	a.m.				
	a.m.				
	p.m.				
	p.m.				

Blood Pressure Log

Month:_____   Week Starting:_____

Time		Blood Pressure		Heart Rate (Pulse Per Minute)	Notes e.g. Medication Change, Activities.
		Systolic (Upper #)	Diastolic (Lower #)		
Monday	a.m.				
	a.m.				
	p.m.				
	p.m.				
Tuesday	a.m.				
	a.m.				
	p.m.				
	p.m.				
Wednesday	a.m.				
	a.m.				
	p.m.				
	p.m.				
Thursday	a.m.				
	a.m.				
	p.m.				
	p.m.				
Friday	a.m.				
	a.m.				
	p.m.				
	p.m.				
Saturday	a.m.				
	a.m.				
	p.m.				
	p.m.				
Sunday	a.m.				
	a.m.				
	p.m.				
	p.m.				

Blood Pressure Log

Month:_____   Week Starting:_____

Time		Blood Pressure		Heart Rate (Pulse Per Minute)	Notes e.g. Medication Change, Activities.
		Systolic (Upper #)	Diastolic (Lower #)		
Monday	a.m.				
Monday	a.m.				
Monday	p.m.				
Monday	p.m.				
Tuesday	a.m.				
Tuesday	a.m.				
Tuesday	p.m.				
Tuesday	p.m.				
Wednesday	a.m.				
Wednesday	a.m.				
Wednesday	p.m.				
Wednesday	p.m.				
Thursday	a.m.				
Thursday	a.m.				
Thursday	p.m.				
Thursday	p.m.				
Friday	a.m.				
Friday	a.m.				
Friday	p.m.				
Friday	p.m.				
Saturday	a.m.				
Saturday	a.m.				
Saturday	p.m.				
Saturday	p.m.				
Sunday	a.m.				
Sunday	a.m.				
Sunday	p.m.				
Sunday	p.m.				

Blood Pressure Log

Month:_____   Week Starting:_____

Time		Blood Pressure		Heart Rate (Pulse Per Minute)	Notes e.g. Medication Change, Activities.
		Systolic (Upper #)	Diastolic (Lower #)		
Monday	a.m.				
	a.m.				
	p.m.				
	p.m.				
Tuesday	a.m.				
	a.m.				
	p.m.				
	p.m.				
Wednesday	a.m.				
	a.m.				
	p.m.				
	p.m.				
Thursday	a.m.				
	a.m.				
	p.m.				
	p.m.				
Friday	a.m.				
	a.m.				
	p.m.				
	p.m.				
Saturday	a.m.				
	a.m.				
	p.m.				
	p.m.				
Sunday	a.m.				
	a.m.				
	p.m.				
	p.m.				

Blood Pressure Log

Month:_____   Week Starting:_____

Time	Blood Pressure		Heart Rate (Pulse Per Minute)	Notes e.g. Medication Change, Activities.
	Systolic (Upper #)	Diastolic (Lower #)		
Monday a.m.				
a.m.				
p.m.				
p.m.				
Tuesday a.m.				
a.m.				
p.m.				
p.m.				
Wednesday a.m.				
a.m.				
p.m.				
p.m.				
Thursday a.m.				
a.m.				
p.m.				
p.m.				
Friday a.m.				
a.m.				
p.m.				
p.m.				
Saturday a.m.				
a.m.				
p.m.				
p.m.				
Sunday a.m.				
a.m.				
p.m.				
p.m.				

Blood Pressure Log

Month:_____   Week Starting:_____

Time		Blood Pressure		Heart Rate (Pulse Per Minute)	Notes e.g. Medication Change, Activities.
		Systolic (Upper #)	Diastolic (Lower #)		
Monday	a.m.				
	a.m.				
	p.m.				
	p.m.				
Tuesday	a.m.				
	a.m.				
	p.m.				
	p.m.				
Wednesday	a.m.				
	a.m.				
	p.m.				
	p.m.				
Thursday	a.m.				
	a.m.				
	p.m.				
	p.m.				
Friday	a.m.				
	a.m.				
	p.m.				
	p.m.				
Saturday	a.m.				
	a.m.				
	p.m.				
	p.m.				
Sunday	a.m.				
	a.m.				
	p.m.				
	p.m.				

Blood Pressure Log

Month:_____   Week Starting:_____

Time	Blood Pressure		Heart Rate (Pulse Per Minute)	Notes e.g. Medication Change, Activities.
	Systolic (Upper #)	Diastolic (Lower #)		
Monday a.m.				
a.m.				
p.m.				
p.m.				
Tuesday a.m.				
a.m.				
p.m.				
p.m.				
Wednesday a.m.				
a.m.				
p.m.				
p.m.				
Thursday a.m.				
a.m.				
p.m.				
p.m.				
Friday a.m.				
a.m.				
p.m.				
p.m.				
Saturday a.m.				
a.m.				
p.m.				
p.m.				
Sunday a.m.				
a.m.				
p.m.				
p.m.				

Blood Pressure Log

Month:_____   Week Starting:_____

Time		Blood Pressure		Heart Rate (Pulse Per Minute)	Notes e.g. Medication Change, Activities.
		Systolic (Upper #)	Diastolic (Lower #)		
Monday	a.m.				
	a.m.				
	p.m.				
	p.m.				
Tuesday	a.m.				
	a.m.				
	p.m.				
	p.m.				
Wednesday	a.m.				
	a.m.				
	p.m.				
	p.m.				
Thursday	a.m.				
	a.m.				
	p.m.				
	p.m.				
Friday	a.m.				
	a.m.				
	p.m.				
	p.m.				
Saturday	a.m.				
	a.m.				
	p.m.				
	p.m.				
Sunday	a.m.				
	a.m.				
	p.m.				
	p.m.				

Blood Pressure Log

Month:_____   Week Starting:_____

Time	Blood Pressure		Heart Rate (Pulse Per Minute)	Notes e.g. Medication Change, Activities.
	Systolic (Upper #)	Diastolic (Lower #)		
Monday a.m.				
a.m.				
p.m.				
p.m.				
Tuesday a.m.				
a.m.				
p.m.				
p.m.				
Wednesday a.m.				
a.m.				
p.m.				
p.m.				
Thursday a.m.				
a.m.				
p.m.				
p.m.				
Friday a.m.				
a.m.				
p.m.				
p.m.				
Saturday a.m.				
a.m.				
p.m.				
p.m.				
Sunday a.m.				
a.m.				
p.m.				
p.m.				

Blood Pressure Log

Month:_____   Week Starting:_____

Time		Blood Pressure		Heart Rate (Pulse Per Minute)	Notes e.g. Medication Change, Activities.
		Systolic (Upper #)	Diastolic (Lower #)		
Monday	a.m.				
	a.m.				
	p.m.				
	p.m.				
Tuesday	a.m.				
	a.m.				
	p.m.				
	p.m.				
Wednesday	a.m.				
	a.m.				
	p.m.				
	p.m.				
Thursday	a.m.				
	a.m.				
	p.m.				
	p.m.				
Friday	a.m.				
	a.m.				
	p.m.				
	p.m.				
Saturday	a.m.				
	a.m.				
	p.m.				
	p.m.				
Sunday	a.m.				
	a.m.				
	p.m.				
	p.m.				

Blood Pressure Log

Month:_____   Week Starting:_____

Time		Blood Pressure		Heart Rate (Pulse Per Minute)	Notes e.g. Medication Change, Activities.
		Systolic (Upper #)	Diastolic (Lower #)		
Monday	a.m.				
	a.m.				
	p.m.				
	p.m.				
Tuesday	a.m.				
	a.m.				
	p.m.				
	p.m.				
Wednesday	a.m.				
	a.m.				
	p.m.				
	p.m.				
Thursday	a.m.				
	a.m.				
	p.m.				
	p.m.				
Friday	a.m.				
	a.m.				
	p.m.				
	p.m.				
Saturday	a.m.				
	a.m.				
	p.m.				
	p.m.				
Sunday	a.m.				
	a.m.				
	p.m.				
	p.m.				

Blood Pressure Log

Month:_____   Week Starting:_____

Time		Blood Pressure		Heart Rate (Pulse Per Minute)	Notes e.g. Medication Change, Activities.
		Systolic (Upper #)	Diastolic (Lower #)		
Monday	a.m.				
	a.m.				
	p.m.				
	p.m.				
Tuesday	a.m.				
	a.m.				
	p.m.				
	p.m.				
Wednesday	a.m.				
	a.m.				
	p.m.				
	p.m.				
Thursday	a.m.				
	a.m.				
	p.m.				
	p.m.				
Friday	a.m.				
	a.m.				
	p.m.				
	p.m.				
Saturday	a.m.				
	a.m.				
	p.m.				
	p.m.				
Sunday	a.m.				
	a.m.				
	p.m.				
	p.m.				

Blood Pressure Log

Month:_____   Week Starting:_____

Time		Blood Pressure		Heart Rate (Pulse Per Minute)	Notes e.g. Medication Change, Activities.
		Systolic (Upper #)	Diastolic (Lower #)		
Monday	a.m.				
	a.m.				
	p.m.				
	p.m.				
Tuesday	a.m.				
	a.m.				
	p.m.				
	p.m.				
Wednesday	a.m.				
	a.m.				
	p.m.				
	p.m.				
Thursday	a.m.				
	a.m.				
	p.m.				
	p.m.				
Friday	a.m.				
	a.m.				
	p.m.				
	p.m.				
Saturday	a.m.				
	a.m.				
	p.m.				
	p.m.				
Sunday	a.m.				
	a.m.				
	p.m.				
	p.m.				

Blood Pressure Log

Month:_____   Week Starting:_____

Time		Blood Pressure		Heart Rate (Pulse Per Minute)	Notes e.g. Medication Change, Activities.
		Systolic (Upper #)	Diastolic (Lower #)		
Monday	a.m.				
	a.m.				
	p.m.				
	p.m.				
Tuesday	a.m.				
	a.m.				
	p.m.				
	p.m.				
Wednesday	a.m.				
	a.m.				
	p.m.				
	p.m.				
Thursday	a.m.				
	a.m.				
	p.m.				
	p.m.				
Friday	a.m.				
	a.m.				
	p.m.				
	p.m.				
Saturday	a.m.				
	a.m.				
	p.m.				
	p.m.				
Sunday	a.m.				
	a.m.				
	p.m.				
	p.m.				

Blood Pressure Log

Month:_____   Week Starting:_____

Time		Blood Pressure		Heart Rate (Pulse Per Minute)	Notes e.g. Medication Change, Activities.
		Systolic (Upper #)	Diastolic (Lower #)		
Monday	a.m.				
	a.m.				
	p.m.				
	p.m.				
Tuesday	a.m.				
	a.m.				
	p.m.				
	p.m.				
Wednesday	a.m.				
	a.m.				
	p.m.				
	p.m.				
Thursday	a.m.				
	a.m.				
	p.m.				
	p.m.				
Friday	a.m.				
	a.m.				
	p.m.				
	p.m.				
Saturday	a.m.				
	a.m.				
	p.m.				
	p.m.				
Sunday	a.m.				
	a.m.				
	p.m.				
	p.m.				

Blood Pressure Log

Month:_____   Week Starting:_____

| Time | Blood Pressure | | Heart Rate (Pulse Per Minute) | Notes e.g. Medication Change, Activities. |
	Systolic (Upper #)	Diastolic (Lower #)		
Monday a.m.				
a.m.				
p.m.				
p.m.				
Tuesday a.m.				
a.m.				
p.m.				
p.m.				
Wednesday a.m.				
a.m.				
p.m.				
p.m.				
Thursday a.m.				
a.m.				
p.m.				
p.m.				
Friday a.m.				
a.m.				
p.m.				
p.m.				
Saturday a.m.				
a.m.				
p.m.				
p.m.				
Sunday a.m.				
a.m.				
p.m.				
p.m.				

Blood Pressure Log

Month:_____   Week Starting:_____

Time	Blood Pressure		Heart Rate (Pulse Per Minute)	Notes e.g. Medication Change, Activities.
	Systolic (Upper #)	Diastolic (Lower #)		
Monday a.m.				
a.m.				
p.m.				
p.m.				
Tuesday a.m.				
a.m.				
p.m.				
p.m.				
Wednesday a.m.				
a.m.				
p.m.				
p.m.				
Thursday a.m.				
a.m.				
p.m.				
p.m.				
Friday a.m.				
a.m.				
p.m.				
p.m.				
Saturday a.m.				
a.m.				
p.m.				
p.m.				
Sunday a.m.				
a.m.				
p.m.				
p.m.				

Blood Pressure Log

Month:_____   Week Starting:_____

Time	Blood Pressure		Heart Rate (Pulse Per Minute)	Notes e.g. Medication Change, Activities.
	Systolic (Upper #)	Diastolic (Lower #)		
Monday a.m.				
a.m.				
p.m.				
p.m.				
Tuesday a.m.				
a.m.				
p.m.				
p.m.				
Wednesday a.m.				
a.m.				
p.m.				
p.m.				
Thursday a.m.				
a.m.				
p.m.				
p.m.				
Friday a.m.				
a.m.				
p.m.				
p.m.				
Saturday a.m.				
a.m.				
p.m.				
p.m.				
Sunday a.m.				
a.m.				
p.m.				
p.m.				

Blood Pressure Log

Month:_____   Week Starting:_____

Time		Blood Pressure		Heart Rate (Pulse Per Minute)	Notes e.g. Medication Change, Activities.
		Systolic (Upper #)	Diastolic (Lower #)		
Monday	a.m.				
	a.m.				
	p.m.				
	p.m.				
Tuesday	a.m.				
	a.m.				
	p.m.				
	p.m.				
Wednesday	a.m.				
	a.m.				
	p.m.				
	p.m.				
Thursday	a.m.				
	a.m.				
	p.m.				
	p.m.				
Friday	a.m.				
	a.m.				
	p.m.				
	p.m.				
Saturday	a.m.				
	a.m.				
	p.m.				
	p.m.				
Sunday	a.m.				
	a.m.				
	p.m.				
	p.m.				

Blood Pressure Log

Month:_____   Week Starting:_____

Time		Blood Pressure		Heart Rate (Pulse Per Minute)	Notes e.g. Medication Change, Activities.
		Systolic (Upper #)	Diastolic (Lower #)		
Monday	a.m.				
	a.m.				
	p.m.				
	p.m.				
Tuesday	a.m.				
	a.m.				
	p.m.				
	p.m.				
Wednesday	a.m.				
	a.m.				
	p.m.				
	p.m.				
Thursday	a.m.				
	a.m.				
	p.m.				
	p.m.				
Friday	a.m.				
	a.m.				
	p.m.				
	p.m.				
Saturday	a.m.				
	a.m.				
	p.m.				
	p.m.				
Sunday	a.m.				
	a.m.				
	p.m.				
	p.m.				

Blood Pressure Log

Month:_____   Week Starting:_____

Time		Blood Pressure		Heart Rate (Pulse Per Minute)	Notes e.g. Medication Change, Activities.
		Systolic (Upper #)	Diastolic (Lower #)		
Monday	a.m.				
	a.m.				
	p.m.				
	p.m.				
Tuesday	a.m.				
	a.m.				
	p.m.				
	p.m.				
Wednesday	a.m.				
	a.m.				
	p.m.				
	p.m.				
Thursday	a.m.				
	a.m.				
	p.m.				
	p.m.				
Friday	a.m.				
	a.m.				
	p.m.				
	p.m.				
Saturday	a.m.				
	a.m.				
	p.m.				
	p.m.				
Sunday	a.m.				
	a.m.				
	p.m.				
	p.m.				

Blood Pressure Log

Month:_____   Week Starting:_____

Time	Blood Pressure		Heart Rate (Pulse Per Minute)	Notes e.g. Medication Change, Activities.
	Systolic (Upper #)	Diastolic (Lower #)		
Monday a.m.				
a.m.				
p.m.				
p.m.				
Tuesday a.m.				
a.m.				
p.m.				
p.m.				
Wednesday a.m.				
a.m.				
p.m.				
p.m.				
Thursday a.m.				
a.m.				
p.m.				
p.m.				
Friday a.m.				
a.m.				
p.m.				
p.m.				
Saturday a.m.				
a.m.				
p.m.				
p.m.				
Sunday a.m.				
a.m.				
p.m.				
p.m.				

Blood Pressure Log

Month:_____   Week Starting:_____

Time		Blood Pressure		Heart Rate (Pulse Per Minute)	Notes e.g. Medication Change, Activities.
		Systolic (Upper #)	Diastolic (Lower #)		
Monday	a.m.				
	a.m.				
	p.m.				
	p.m.				
Tuesday	a.m.				
	a.m.				
	p.m.				
	p.m.				
Wednesday	a.m.				
	a.m.				
	p.m.				
	p.m.				
Thursday	a.m.				
	a.m.				
	p.m.				
	p.m.				
Friday	a.m.				
	a.m.				
	p.m.				
	p.m.				
Saturday	a.m.				
	a.m.				
	p.m.				
	p.m.				
Sunday	a.m.				
	a.m.				
	p.m.				
	p.m.				

Blood Pressure Log

Month:_____   Week Starting:_____

Time		Blood Pressure		Heart Rate (Pulse Per Minute)	Notes e.g. Medication Change, Activities.
		Systolic (Upper #)	Diastolic (Lower #)		
Monday	a.m.				
	a.m.				
	p.m.				
	p.m.				
Tuesday	a.m.				
	a.m.				
	p.m.				
	p.m.				
Wednesday	a.m.				
	a.m.				
	p.m.				
	p.m.				
Thursday	a.m.				
	a.m.				
	p.m.				
	p.m.				
Friday	a.m.				
	a.m.				
	p.m.				
	p.m.				
Saturday	a.m.				
	a.m.				
	p.m.				
	p.m.				
Sunday	a.m.				
	a.m.				
	p.m.				
	p.m.				

Blood Pressure Log

Month:_____   Week Starting:_____

Time	Blood Pressure		Heart Rate (Pulse Per Minute)	Notes e.g. Medication Change, Activities.
	Systolic (Upper #)	Diastolic (Lower #)		
Monday a.m.				
a.m.				
p.m.				
p.m.				
Tuesday a.m.				
a.m.				
p.m.				
p.m.				
Wednesday a.m.				
a.m.				
p.m.				
p.m.				
Thursday a.m.				
a.m.				
p.m.				
p.m.				
Friday a.m.				
a.m.				
p.m.				
p.m.				
Saturday a.m.				
a.m.				
p.m.				
p.m.				
Sunday a.m.				
a.m.				
p.m.				
p.m.				

Blood Pressure Log

Month:_____   Week Starting:_____

Time		Blood Pressure		Heart Rate (Pulse Per Minute)	Notes e.g. Medication Change, Activities.
		Systolic (Upper #)	Diastolic (Lower #)		
Monday	a.m.				
	a.m.				
	p.m.				
	p.m.				
Tuesday	a.m.				
	a.m.				
	p.m.				
	p.m.				
Wednesday	a.m.				
	a.m.				
	p.m.				
	p.m.				
Thursday	a.m.				
	a.m.				
	p.m.				
	p.m.				
Friday	a.m.				
	a.m.				
	p.m.				
	p.m.				
Saturday	a.m.				
	a.m.				
	p.m.				
	p.m.				
Sunday	a.m.				
	a.m.				
	p.m.				
	p.m.				

Blood Pressure Log

Month:_____   Week Starting:_____

Time		Blood Pressure		Heart Rate (Pulse Per Minute)	Notes e.g. Medication Change, Activities.
		Systolic (Upper #)	Diastolic (Lower #)		
Monday	a.m.				
	a.m.				
	p.m.				
	p.m.				
Tuesday	a.m.				
	a.m.				
	p.m.				
	p.m.				
Wednesday	a.m.				
	a.m.				
	p.m.				
	p.m.				
Thursday	a.m.				
	a.m.				
	p.m.				
	p.m.				
Friday	a.m.				
	a.m.				
	p.m.				
	p.m.				
Saturday	a.m.				
	a.m.				
	p.m.				
	p.m.				
Sunday	a.m.				
	a.m.				
	p.m.				
	p.m.				

Blood Pressure Log

Month:_____   Week Starting:_____

Time	Blood Pressure		Heart Rate (Pulse Per Minute)	Notes e.g. Medication Change, Activities.
	Systolic (Upper #)	Diastolic (Lower #)		
Monday a.m.				
a.m.				
p.m.				
p.m.				
Tuesday a.m.				
a.m.				
p.m.				
p.m.				
Wednesday a.m.				
a.m.				
p.m.				
p.m.				
Thursday a.m.				
a.m.				
p.m.				
p.m.				
Friday a.m.				
a.m.				
p.m.				
p.m.				
Saturday a.m.				
a.m.				
p.m.				
p.m.				
Sunday a.m.				
a.m.				
p.m.				
p.m.				

Blood Pressure Log

Month:_____   Week Starting:_____

Time	Blood Pressure		Heart Rate (Pulse Per Minute)	Notes e.g. Medication Change, Activities.
	Systolic (Upper #)	Diastolic (Lower #)		
Monday a.m.				
a.m.				
p.m.				
p.m.				
Tuesday a.m.				
a.m.				
p.m.				
p.m.				
Wednesday a.m.				
a.m.				
p.m.				
p.m.				
Thursday a.m.				
a.m.				
p.m.				
p.m.				
Friday a.m.				
a.m.				
p.m.				
p.m.				
Saturday a.m.				
a.m.				
p.m.				
p.m.				
Sunday a.m.				
a.m.				
p.m.				
p.m.				

Blood Pressure Log

Month:_____   Week Starting:_____

Time		Blood Pressure		Heart Rate (Pulse Per Minute)	Notes e.g. Medication Change, Activities.
		Systolic (Upper #)	Diastolic (Lower #)		
Monday	a.m.				
	a.m.				
	p.m.				
	p.m.				
Tuesday	a.m.				
	a.m.				
	p.m.				
	p.m.				
Wednesday	a.m.				
	a.m.				
	p.m.				
	p.m.				
Thursday	a.m.				
	a.m.				
	p.m.				
	p.m.				
Friday	a.m.				
	a.m.				
	p.m.				
	p.m.				
Saturday	a.m.				
	a.m.				
	p.m.				
	p.m.				
Sunday	a.m.				
	a.m.				
	p.m.				
	p.m.				

Blood Pressure Log

Month:_____   Week Starting:_____

Time	Blood Pressure		Heart Rate (Pulse Per Minute)	Notes e.g. Medication Change, Activities.
	Systolic (Upper #)	Diastolic (Lower #)		
Monday a.m.				
a.m.				
p.m.				
p.m.				
Tuesday a.m.				
a.m.				
p.m.				
p.m.				
Wednesday a.m.				
a.m.				
p.m.				
p.m.				
Thursday a.m.				
a.m.				
p.m.				
p.m.				
Friday a.m.				
a.m.				
p.m.				
p.m.				
Saturday a.m.				
a.m.				
p.m.				
p.m.				
Sunday a.m.				
a.m.				
p.m.				
p.m.				

Blood Pressure Log

Month:_____   Week Starting:_____

Time	Blood Pressure		Heart Rate (Pulse Per Minute)	Notes e.g. Medication Change, Activities.
	Systolic (Upper #)	Diastolic (Lower #)		
Monday a.m.				
a.m.				
p.m.				
p.m.				
Tuesday a.m.				
a.m.				
p.m.				
p.m.				
Wednesday a.m.				
a.m.				
p.m.				
p.m.				
Thursday a.m.				
a.m.				
p.m.				
p.m.				
Friday a.m.				
a.m.				
p.m.				
p.m.				
Saturday a.m.				
a.m.				
p.m.				
p.m.				
Sunday a.m.				
a.m.				
p.m.				
p.m.				

Blood Pressure Log

Month:_____   Week Starting:_____

Time		Blood Pressure		Heart Rate (Pulse Per Minute)	Notes e.g. Medication Change, Activities.
		Systolic (Upper #)	Diastolic (Lower #)		
Monday	a.m.				
	a.m.				
	p.m.				
	p.m.				
Tuesday	a.m.				
	a.m.				
	p.m.				
	p.m.				
Wednesday	a.m.				
	a.m.				
	p.m.				
	p.m.				
Thursday	a.m.				
	a.m.				
	p.m.				
	p.m.				
Friday	a.m.				
	a.m.				
	p.m.				
	p.m.				
Saturday	a.m.				
	a.m.				
	p.m.				
	p.m.				
Sunday	a.m.				
	a.m.				
	p.m.				
	p.m.				

Blood Pressure Log

Month:_____   Week Starting:_____

Time	Blood Pressure		Heart Rate (Pulse Per Minute)	Notes e.g. Medication Change, Activities.
	Systolic (Upper #)	Diastolic (Lower #)		
Monday a.m.				
a.m.				
p.m.				
p.m.				
Tuesday a.m.				
a.m.				
p.m.				
p.m.				
Wednesday a.m.				
a.m.				
p.m.				
p.m.				
Thursday a.m.				
a.m.				
p.m.				
p.m.				
Friday a.m.				
a.m.				
p.m.				
p.m.				
Saturday a.m.				
a.m.				
p.m.				
p.m.				
Sunday a.m.				
a.m.				
p.m.				
p.m.				

Blood Pressure Log

Month:_____   Week Starting:_____

Time	Blood Pressure		Heart Rate (Pulse Per Minute)	Notes e.g. Medication Change, Activities.
	Systolic (Upper #)	Diastolic (Lower #)		
Monday a.m.				
a.m.				
p.m.				
p.m.				
Tuesday a.m.				
a.m.				
p.m.				
p.m.				
Wednesday a.m.				
a.m.				
p.m.				
p.m.				
Thursday a.m.				
a.m.				
p.m.				
p.m.				
Friday a.m.				
a.m.				
p.m.				
p.m.				
Saturday a.m.				
a.m.				
p.m.				
p.m.				
Sunday a.m.				
a.m.				
p.m.				
p.m.				

Blood Pressure Log

Month:_____   Week Starting:_____

Time	Blood Pressure		Heart Rate (Pulse Per Minute)	Notes e.g. Medication Change, Activities.
	Systolic (Upper #)	Diastolic (Lower #)		
Monday a.m.				
a.m.				
p.m.				
p.m.				
Tuesday a.m.				
a.m.				
p.m.				
p.m.				
Wednesday a.m.				
a.m.				
p.m.				
p.m.				
Thursday a.m.				
a.m.				
p.m.				
p.m.				
Friday a.m.				
a.m.				
p.m.				
p.m.				
Saturday a.m.				
a.m.				
p.m.				
p.m.				
Sunday a.m.				
a.m.				
p.m.				
p.m.				

Blood Pressure Log

Month:_____   Week Starting:_____

Time	Blood Pressure		Heart Rate (Pulse Per Minute)	Notes e.g. Medication Change, Activities.
	Systolic (Upper #)	Diastolic (Lower #)		
Monday a.m.				
a.m.				
p.m.				
p.m.				
Tuesday a.m.				
a.m.				
p.m.				
p.m.				
Wednesday a.m.				
a.m.				
p.m.				
p.m.				
Thursday a.m.				
a.m.				
p.m.				
p.m.				
Friday a.m.				
a.m.				
p.m.				
p.m.				
Saturday a.m.				
a.m.				
p.m.				
p.m.				
Sunday a.m.				
a.m.				
p.m.				
p.m.				

Blood Pressure Log

Month:_____   Week Starting:_____

Time	Blood Pressure		Heart Rate (Pulse Per Minute)	Notes e.g. Medication Change, Activities.
	Systolic (Upper #)	Diastolic (Lower #)		
Monday a.m.				
a.m.				
p.m.				
p.m.				
Tuesday a.m.				
a.m.				
p.m.				
p.m.				
Wednesday a.m.				
a.m.				
p.m.				
p.m.				
Thursday a.m.				
a.m.				
p.m.				
p.m.				
Friday a.m.				
a.m.				
p.m.				
p.m.				
Saturday a.m.				
a.m.				
p.m.				
p.m.				
Sunday a.m.				
a.m.				
p.m.				
p.m.				

Blood Pressure Log

Month:_____   Week Starting:_____

Time		Blood Pressure		Heart Rate (Pulse Per Minute)	Notes e.g. Medication Change, Activities.
		Systolic (Upper #)	Diastolic (Lower #)		
Monday	a.m.				
	a.m.				
	p.m.				
	p.m.				
Tuesday	a.m.				
	a.m.				
	p.m.				
	p.m.				
Wednesday	a.m.				
	a.m.				
	p.m.				
	p.m.				
Thursday	a.m.				
	a.m.				
	p.m.				
	p.m.				
Friday	a.m.				
	a.m.				
	p.m.				
	p.m.				
Saturday	a.m.				
	a.m.				
	p.m.				
	p.m.				
Sunday	a.m.				
	a.m.				
	p.m.				
	p.m.				

Blood Pressure Log

Month:_____   Week Starting:_____

Time		Blood Pressure		Heart Rate (Pulse Per Minute)	Notes e.g. Medication Change, Activities.
		Systolic (Upper #)	Diastolic (Lower #)		
Monday	a.m.				
	a.m.				
	p.m.				
	p.m.				
Tuesday	a.m.				
	a.m.				
	p.m.				
	p.m.				
Wednesday	a.m.				
	a.m.				
	p.m.				
	p.m.				
Thursday	a.m.				
	a.m.				
	p.m.				
	p.m.				
Friday	a.m.				
	a.m.				
	p.m.				
	p.m.				
Saturday	a.m.				
	a.m.				
	p.m.				
	p.m.				
Sunday	a.m.				
	a.m.				
	p.m.				
	p.m.